You've Got the Power

CHOOSE TO SHINE

every day

be the BEST version of ★you

YOU'RE-DOING Great

Believe in Yourself

POSITIVE MIND

SMILE everyday

I am capable

you're AMAZING

-STAY- POSITIVE

YES YOU CAN

FOCUS ON THE GOOD

GOOD VIBES

clean your MIND

FOLLOW YOUR HEART

BE Bold

you are loved

You Got This!

be happy ♥

TREAT yourself

Proud OF myself

CHASE Goals

be Brave

you're LOVED

Kindness MATTERS

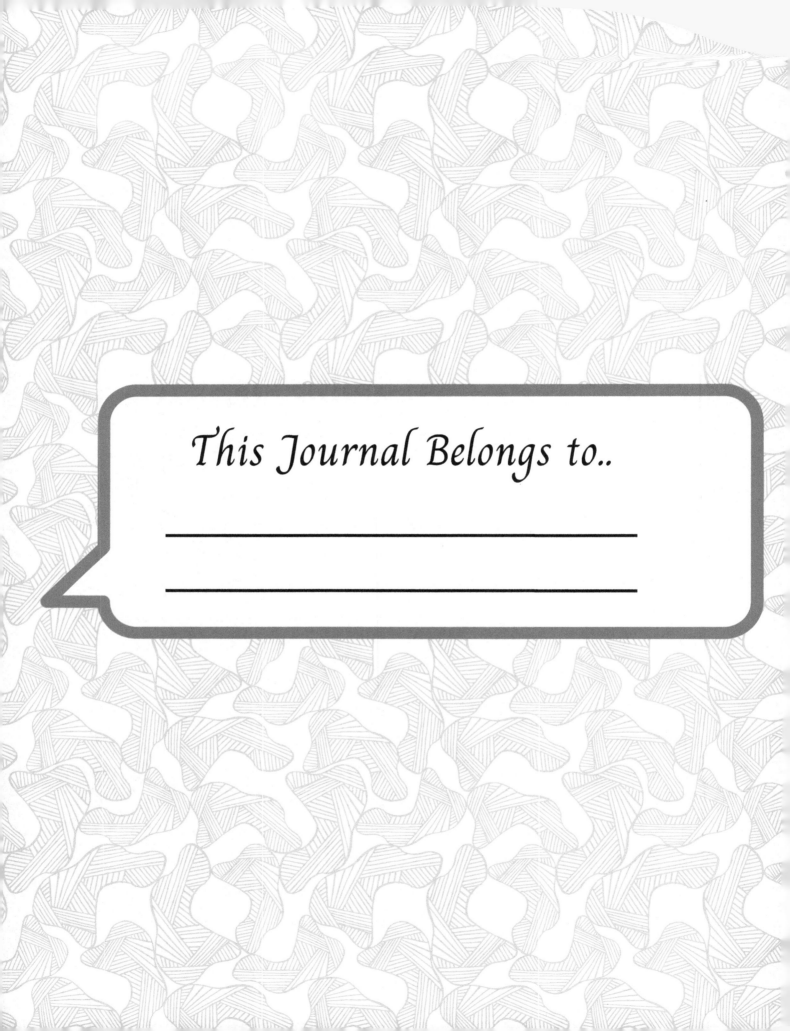

This Journal Belongs to..

_____

_____

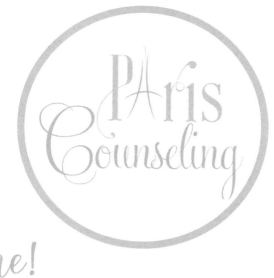

Well hi there!

Welcome! Come on in! Have a seat, grab something to sip on and let's get down to business.

How are you? No, I mean, how are you, really? I've been feeling a little defeated lately. Do you ever feel like no matter what you do, you just can't seem to feel settled? Comfortable in your skin? Fulfilled? Me too. I think I am mostly just trying to keep my head above water. Ever wonder why? There are so many reasons, and most of them aren't your fault. But, even if things aren't necessarily our fault, we can still take control, and it IS our job to help ourselves be better. That is where this journal comes in!

Do you currently journal, or have you ever kept a journal? The benefits of keeping a journal such as this one include long-term improvements in mood, decreased stress, and a reduction in depressive symptoms. It actually can also help improve physical symptoms. Don't take our word for it; a study in 2013 in New Zealand found that adults who participated in journalling healed from physical injury faster than those in the control group. In fact, 76% of the participants in the study had recovered fully in two weeks from their physical ailments while only 42% of the control group had improved symptoms (Rodriguez, 2013). The researcher attributed this to the reduction of stress in the body, due to the processing of emotions that occurs when one journals their feelings.

This journal will also serve as a form of self-discovery. We cannot get to the bottom of what is keeping us from being our absolute healthiest without a little mental self-exploration. Get ready friends; feeling your best is our ultimate goal!

Why do You Need This Activity Each Day?

Repeat after me: I am worth the time it takes to complete these pages. Say it again. One more time. We know you are busy; life is busy! But we also know that until you take time for yourself, you aren't doing yourself justice. We aren't asking for two hours of your day, or even one hour (but wouldn't that be amazing?!). We would love it if you could take 15 minutes to sit down with this journal every day and just stop: stop the noise, stop your busy thoughts, and focus on you. You matter, you are worth it, and you are important. Since you are important, so is your self-care. Read this paragraph over and over until you hear it in your soul.

Raise your hand if you are ready to give yourself the time you deserve! Higher! Come on now, no one is watching! Throw those hands in the air! Ok put them down you look ridiculous. I'M KIDDING I'M KIDDING! You look great! Walk around like that! It's good for circulation and keeps your fingers looking less like sausages. Blood flow is important ;)
Ok. Put them down whenever you feel like it.

Oh. And it doesn't matter when you start this baby; January 1, February 27th, March 31, August 28th, September 18th, or October 8th. It doesn't matter what season you're in or what cycle of the moon is waxing or waning; anytime is the right time! We have given you 28 days of specific journaling. It takes 28 days to form a habit; our hope is that after you stick to these 28 days, you will not only see the benefit to your well-being, but you will also create a new and lovely habit.

Some days are worse than others, right? This is true for everyone. When you are really struggling, as we all do from time to time, check out the Struggle Bus section on Page 105. This section is a wonderful tool for those days when we just aren't sure how the sun is going to rise again. It focuses on the cognitive behavioral therapy model and allows you to really process what is happening and how you are handling it. It's good stuff. You can use it in addition to a regular daily journal entry or simply on its own; you do you, boo.

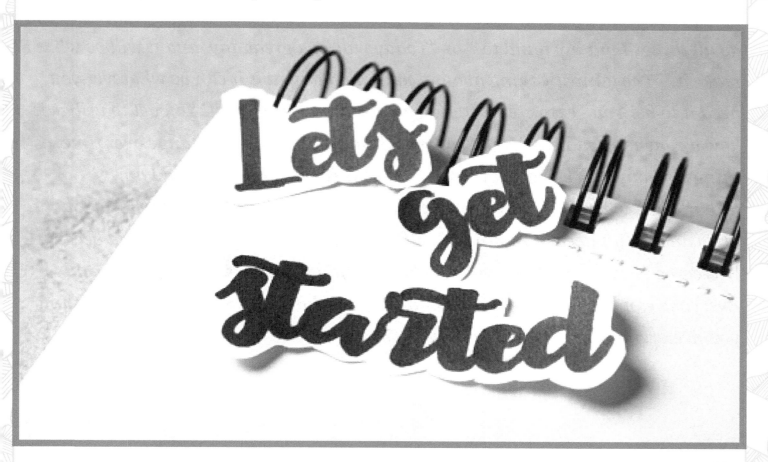

Tools, Terms and Techniques

What's your mantra?

Do you have a mantra? Are you wondering what a mantra is?

You wouldn't be alone. A mantra has traditionally been a short sound or phrase repeated during meditation or prayer to keep your mind and body focused on the moment. In today's day and age, the term mantra has also been used to describe a self-affirming phrase you use daily to remind yourself of what is important to you. A personal mantra might give you strength to get through a tough day, such as "I am brave and ready for this challenge." It might be a tool to remind yourself "I can do all things I put my mind to," or "Today will be a great day, and it will be what I make it." The fantastic thing about a personal mantra is it can be whatever you need it to be! You get to create it! You get to keep it to yourself! You get to utilize it how and when you need to! It's yours and yours alone. It can change over time, as things in your life change. My mantra once was "I have worth and I am important," when I wasn't feeling very important in the world. I learned a lot, grew and didn't need to remind myself of that anymore! My new mantra became "I create my own happiness and will keep positive thoughts." Ok, your turn! Everyone can benefit from a daily mantra! Just think of the most important thing you need reminding of right now; you got this.

Thinking Errors

Thinking errors: we all have them. Also called cognitive distortions, thinking errors are irrational thoughts that fuel an unhealthy emotional state. Worry, anxiety, anger, poor mood, and sadness are emotions that can all lead us into a deep downward spiral of irrational thoughts. The good news is, we can learn to catch those thoughts and redirect them! Catching our thinking errors and learning to reframe ourselves is one of the most important steps in becoming emotionally healthy. In this journal, we will ask you to recognize thinking errors, and ask you to reframe these thoughts. You'll soon see just how beneficial this is when practiced every day.

Thought Stopping Techniques

These are techniques used to reframe and erase those thinking errors! These cognitive behavioral therapy techniques are a way to stop unwanted thoughts and replace them with healthy positive thinking. When you catch yourself in a thought you want to stop, you can:

1) Picture a stop sign in your head, and say "Stop!" to yourself.
2) Snap your fingers in front of your nose to get your attention and redirect yourself.
3) Envision yourself catching the negative thought in a butterfly net, and throwing it out the window.

4) Tense all your muscles up at once and hold for 10 seconds before releasing. This gets some of that negative energy out but also stops your negative thought process.

5) Throw on some headphones and turn up your favorite song! Change your thoughts, change your day!

Coping Skills

I would be willing to bet a million alpacas you have heard this term before. Coping skills are techniques to help you manage stressful moments. Let's drop some coping skills right here to give you a quick reference when you need them.

1) *Deep breathing* : There are TONS of breathing techniques to help slow your thoughts and redirect your energy at times of stress. Box breathing is one of my favorites: breath in for four seconds, hold your breath for four seconds, breathe out for four seconds, hold for four seconds. Picture outlining a box in your head as you breathe each time. Breathe in for four seconds, (draw a line upward) hold for four seconds, (draw a line across) breathe out for four seconds, (draw a line down) hold for four seconds (draw a line back across to complete the box). There are physical things happening in your brain when you practice box breathing; it's not just emotional. Breathing this way adds oxygen to your blood and stimulates the vagus nerve, which runs from the brain to the abdomen. This helps turn off your fight or flight response and calms your nervous system.

2) *Make a cup of tea* : Tea is comforting and medicinal. Find your favorite herbal tea and use tea time as a period of relaxation and respite. Stop the business of the day that has you stressed, and take a moment to yourself to regroup.

3) Aromatherapy is a thing; it's science actually. Certain smells activate certain processes in the brain and can ramp you up or slow you down. When you find yourself in an anxious moment, have some soothing lotion or chapstick on hand. Eucalyptus, spearmint, lavender, chamomile, and ylang-ylang are all scents that work to calm the nervous system. Keep some lotion or a candle handy (or whatever vehicle of scent delivery works for you ;).

4) "Regis, I'd like to phone a friend." If you have the time, text or call a friend whom you know is good for a pick-me-up! Don't call Negative Nancy, that's not helpful. Call Happy Helen or Hilarious Hannah- they are sure to redirect anything stressy in your day!

5) Go for a quick walk outside. Do you love nature as we do? Hit your local park, look at the green space, and breathe deep, friend. The trees really do hear your need for clarity, and nature responds with nurturing magic.

These aren't the only coping skills, obviously; but you get the idea. Do something you know will relieve some stress and put you back on the path to positive thinking.

For the next 28 days, each journal entry will have a list of questions for you to answer. These questions are helpful in gauging where your mindset is and where you would like it to be. It serves as a redirect and can be a valuable tool in learning more about you. Self-awareness is everything; it allows us to identify our good qualities as well as those we would like to change. Without identifying what makes us tick, we will never figure out how best to tock.

Ok-ready for day one? Remember, this works best when you practice this activity every day; however, life is crazy and days are hectic. Pick it up as often as you can; we think you'll see the benefit pretty soon :)

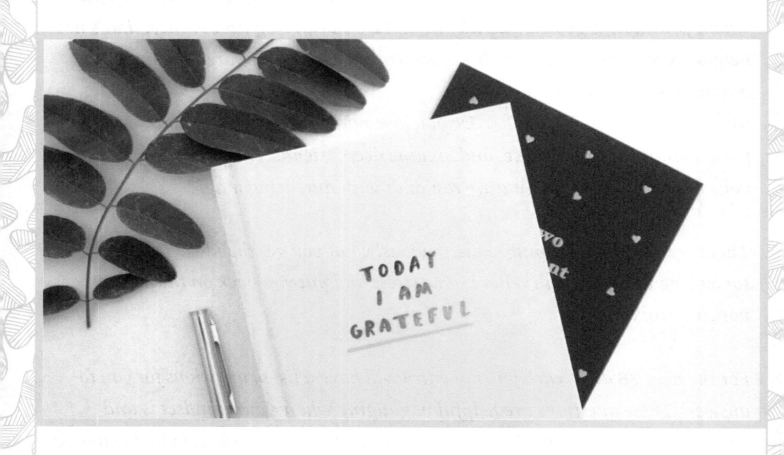

Day One

What's that mantra, friend? Write your mantra here:

_____

_____

Write a little about your day. What was good? What wasn't so good? How did you feel? Sometimes it can be beneficial to keep track of things that happen in life, and then go back and read it next year.If we don't write it down, we forget how far we have come! Tracking your progress can be so encouraging, and let's be real, it's just fun :)

_____

_____

_____

_____

_____

_____

_____

Did you get some good old fashioned exercise?

_____

_____

What have you eaten today that was good for your body and your soul?

_____

_____

Do you think you will have time to meditate/pray/spend 15 minutes quieting your mind? Write down when this fits in your day, and your pledge to yourself to keep this a priority.

_____

_____

List three positive things that happened today:

1) _____

2) _____

3) _____

"Every negative belief weakens the partnership between mind and body."

—Deepak Chopra

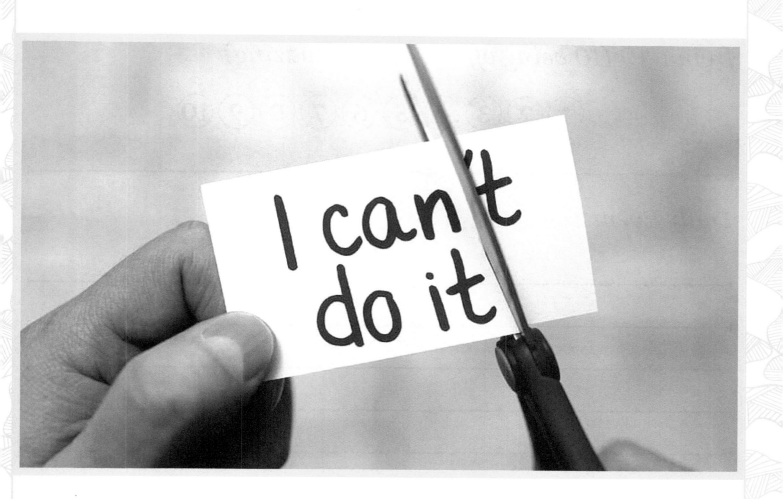

Day Two

Time to write that mantra!

_____

_____

How would you rate how you are feeling today? on a scale from 1-10 (10 being off the charts amazing)

① ② ③ ④ ⑤ ⑥ ⑦ ⑧ ⑨ ⑩

_____

Daily Events:

_____

_____

_____

_____

_____

_____

_____

_____

Ask yourself what is one thing I can do for myself to move me in a healthy direction. This can be emotionally, mentally, physically or spiritually.

_____

_____

_____

List three positive things that happened today:

1) _____

2) _____

3) _____

"If I just offered everybody here a million dollars cash with no strings attached, imagine the excitement and enthusiasm you'd feel. You'd get this money and you're like 'oh man, this is exciting!' Nothing would bother you! But when you wake up in the morning, you don't feel the same way. But waking up in the morning is worth more than a million dollars; how do I know? Because if I said I'll give you a million dollars but you can't wake up tomorrow, none of you would take me up on it. You're getting something more valuable than a million dollars every single day; the first news you get as soon as you open your eyes, start getting excited. Be grateful like you're getting a million dollars."

Gratitude is everything

—Brad Lea

Day Three

You already know-mantra time!

_____

_____

How would you rate how you are feeling today? on a scale from 1-10 (10 being off the charts amazing)

①②③④⑤⑥⑦⑧⑨⑩

If you rated yourself 5 or higher, go get 'em, tiger! See what you can accomplish today! Write those accomplishments down and feel good about it!

If you rated yourself 5 or lower, let's dig in to that.

What is the situation right now occupying your mind?

_____

_____

_____

_____

_____

Are you noticing any physical symptoms? If so, what are they?

_____

_____

_____

_____

Are you noticing any negative thoughts? If so, list them.

_____

_____

_____

_____

Are you able to identify your emotions? (If you are struggling to identify exactly how you are feeling, look at Page 109 to see a list of emotions that we sometimes have difficulty pinpointing.) What emotions are you feeling?

_____

_____

_____

_____

This is a great time to start thinking about thought stopping techniques and coping skills. Let's take a break, let you catch your breath and jot down some notes about your day if you feel like it.

Notes:

_____

_____

_____

_____

_____

_____

_____

_____

Day Four

You guessed it! Mantra:

_____

_____

How would you rate how you are feeling today? on a scale from 1-10 (10 being off the charts amazing)

① ② ③ ④ ⑤ ⑥ ⑦ ⑧ ⑨ ⑩

_____

Daily Events:

_____

_____

_____

_____

_____

_____

_____

Are you currently, or were you aware of your behavior today?
Was it positive or negative? Explain.

_____

_____

_____

_____

If you found yourself stressy, did you use coping skills? What coping skills did you use? If you didn't think to use those skills, what strategies could you have used today? This is a good way to list them and then remind yourself next time.

_____

_____

_____

_____

Were you able to reframe negative thoughts? Tell me more! Yes, I sure did and here's how, or no, and explain why.

_____

_____

_____

_____

_____

_____

Were you able to be present? Explain yes or no and why or why not.

_____

_____

_____

_____

What are some thought stopping techniques you used today, or could use in the future?

_____

_____

_____

_____

Let's evaluate the day. How do you think your day ended as opposed to how it started? Rate your recovery from any negative situations 1-10 (10 being amazing and 1 being lousy). If your day started amazing and finished amazing, high five on that 10/10 day! If you found yourself working hard to reframe and recover, high five on doing the work! Rate your day/recovery here:

①②③④⑤⑥⑦⑧⑨⑩

List three positive things that happened today:

1) _____

2) _____

3) _____

Get some good sleep tonight! Rest up!

"A good laugh and a long sleep are the best cures in the doctor's book."

— Irish proverb

Day Five

Mantra:

_____

_____

Daily Events:

_____

_____

_____

_____

_____

_____

_____

List the emotions you felt:

_____

_____

_____

_____

If you had a negative emotion, were you able to change your emotion?

If yes, great job! If no, explain why?

_____

_____

_____

_____

If you had a negative emotion and were able to change it, did your behavior change?

_____

_____

_____

_____

Please explain the evidence you uncovered to support your reframe.

_____

_____

_____

_____

_____

After evaluating this situation, on a scale from 1-10 (10 being off the charts amazing), how do you think you did helping yourself?

(1)(2)(3)(4)(5)(6)(7)(8)(9)(10)

_____

_____

_____

_____

If you rated how you did with this situation 5 or higher, what did you do that was so effective in helping?

_____

_____

_____

If you rated your handling of the situation 5 or lower, what do you think you could do better next time?

_____

_____

_____

_____

List three positive things that happened today:

1) _____

2) _____

3) _____

"Challenges are what make life interesting; overcoming them is what makes them meaningful."

—Unknown Author

Day Six

Mantra!

_____

_____

Write a little about your day. What was good? What wasn't so good? How did you feel? If we don't write it down, we forget how far we have come! Track your progress!

_____

_____

_____

_____

_____

_____

_____

Did you get some exercise?

_____

What have you eaten today that was good for your body and your soul?

_____

_____

Do you think you will have time to meditate/pray/spend 15 minutes quieting your mind? Write down when this fits in your day, and your pledge to yourself to keep this a priority.

_____

_____

List three positive things that happened today:

1) _____

2) _____

3) _____

Are you having trouble coming up with positive things for today? Did something or someone make you giggle? At any point did you feel relief about something? Did you see a friend, visit a family member, eat a good meal, or play with your pet? These are all rather normal, sometimes mundane things that we take for granted from time to time. Heck, I'm grateful I put one foot in front of the other sometimes!

Day Seven

Time to write that mantra!

_____

_____

How would you rate how you are feeling today? on a scale from 1-10 (10 being off the charts amazing)

①②③④⑤⑥⑦⑧⑨⑩

_____

Daily Events:

_____

_____

_____

_____

_____

_____

_____

_____

Ask yourself what is one thing I can do for myself to move me in a healthy direction. This can be emotionally, mentally, physically or spiritually.

_____

_____

_____

_____

List three positive things that happened today:

1) _____

2) _____

3) _____

Look, I don't know who first said the thing about putting the oxygen mask on yourself first so you can help others, because it kind of annoys me. But, it's true. You have to take care of you, so that you can in turn take care of your family or friends when they need you. That's how this whole thing is supposed to work; we take care of ourselves and take care of each other. So advocate for yourself and your overall health! You deserve it, and your loved ones deserve the best version of you.

Day Eight

Gimme that mantra!

_____

_____

How would you rate how you are feeling today? on a scale from 1-10 (10 being off the charts amazing)

① ② ③ ④ ⑤ ⑥ ⑦ ⑧ ⑨ ⑩

_____

If you rated yourself 5 or higher, nice work! See what you can accomplish today! Write those accomplishments down and feel good about it!

If you rated yourself 5 or lower, let's dig in to that.

What is the situation right now occupying your mind?

_____

_____

_____

Are you noticing any physical symptoms? If so, what are they?

_____

_____

_____

_____

Are you noticing any negative thoughts? If so, list them.

_____

_____

_____

Are you able to identify your emotions? (If you are struggling to identify exactly how you are feeling, look at Page 109 to see a list of emotions that we sometimes have difficulty pinpointing.) What emotions are you feeling?

_____

_____

_____

_____

Hit me with those thought stopping techniques and coping skills. Let's take a break, let you catch your breath and jot down some notes about your day if you feel like it.

Notes:

_____

_____

_____

_____

_____

_____

_____

_____

_____

_____

_____

Day Nine

You guessed it! Mantra:

_____

_____

How would you rate how you are feeling today? on a scale from 1-10 (10 being off the charts amazing)

① ② ③ ④ ⑤ ⑥ ⑦ ⑧ ⑨ ⑩

_____

Daily Events:

_____

_____

_____

_____

_____

_____

_____

_____

Are you currently, or were you aware of your behavior today? Was it positive or negative? Explain.

_____

_____

_____

_____

If you found yourself stressy, did you use coping skills? What coping skills did you use? If you didn't think to use those skills, what strategies could you have used today? This is a good way to list them and then remind yourself next time.

_____

_____

_____

_____

Were you able to reframe negative thoughts? Tell me more! Yes, I sure did and here's how, or no, and explain why.

_____

_____

_____

Were you able to be present? Explain yes or no and why or why not.

What are some thought stopping techniques you used today, or could use in the future?

Let's evaluate the day. How do you think your day ended as opposed to how it started? Rate your recovery from any negative situations 1-10 (10 being amazing and 1 being lousy). If your day started amazing and finished amazing, high five on that 10/10 day! If you found yourself working hard to reframe and recover, high five on doing the work! Rate your day/recovery here:

_____

_____

_____

List three positive things that happened today:

1) _____

2) _____

3) _____

Get some quality shut eye! Good sleep helps us think better the following day, builds our immune systems, improves mood, reduces stress, and keeps our circadian rhythm in balance. I read that Jennifer Lopez never gets less than 8 hours of sleep a night; if it's good enough for J.Lo, it's good enough for us.

Day Ten

Mantra!

_____

_____

Daily Events:

_____

_____

_____

_____

_____

_____

_____

List the emotions you felt:

_____

_____

_____

If you had a negative emotion, were you able to change your emotion?

If yes, great job! If no, explain why?

_____

_____

_____

_____

If you had a negative emotion and were able to change it, did your behavior change?

_____

_____

_____

_____

Please explain the evidence you uncovered to support your reframe.

_____

_____

_____

_____

After evaluating this situation, on a scale from 1-10 (10 being off the charts amazing), how do you think you did helping yourself?

If you rated how you did with this situation 5 or higher, what did you do that was so effective in helping?

If you rated your handling of the situation 5 or lower, what do you think you could do better next time?

List three positive things that happened today:

1) _____

2) _____

3) _____

Do one small thing to make today better than yesterday.

Day Eleven

Mantra!

_____

_____

Daily Events:

_____

_____

_____

_____

_____

_____

_____

List the emotions you felt:

_____

_____

_____

If you had a negative emotion, were you able to change your emotion?

If yes, great job! If no, explain why?

_____

_____

_____

_____

If you had a negative emotion and were able to change it, did your behavior change?

_____

_____

_____

_____

Please explain the evidence you uncovered to support your reframe.

_____

_____

_____

_____

After evaluating this situation, on a scale from 1-10 (10 being off the charts amazing), how do you think you did helping yourself?

_____

_____

_____

_____

If you rated how you did with this situation 5 or higher, what did you do that was so effective in helping?

_____

_____

_____

If you rated your handling of the situation 5 or lower, what do you think you could do better next time?

_____

_____

_____

_____

List three positive things that happened today:

1) _____

2) _____

3) _____

Be mindful. Be grateful. Be positive. Be true. Be kind.

—Roy T. Bennett

Day Twelve

Mantra!

_____

_____

Write a little about your day. What was good? What wasn't so good? How did you feel? If we don't write it down, we forget how far we have come! Track your progress!

_____

_____

_____

_____

_____

_____

_____

_____

Did you get some exercise?

_____

What have you eaten today that was good for your body and your soul?

_____

_____

Do you think you will have time to meditate/pray/spend 15 minutes quieting your mind? Write down when this fits in your day, and your pledge to yourself to keep this a priority.

_____

_____

List three positive things that happened today:

1) _____

2) _____

3) _____

Day Thirteen

Time to write that mantra!

_____

_____

How would you rate how you are feeling today? on a scale from 1-10 (10 being off the charts amazing)

① ② ③ ④ ⑤ ⑥ ⑦ ⑧ ⑨ ⑩

_____

Daily Events:

_____

_____

_____

_____

_____

_____

_____

Ask yourself what is one thing I can do for myself to move me in a healthy direction. This can be emotionally, mentally, physically or spiritually.

_____

_____

_____

List three positive things that happened today:

1) _____

2) _____

3) _____

Let's take just a second to talk about nutrition. What you put in your body can fuel it or destroy it. Eating a diet rich in vegetables and fruits, along with whole grains and good sources of protein can do wonders for your mental clarity as well as your physical health. We highly recommend keeping a food journal if you are feeling sluggish or out of sorts. See what you are eating and if it correlates with physical or emotional symptoms.

You could have some food allergies or sensitivities of which you are unaware. Getting your gut healthy is super important to your emotional health. There is so much new research that shows your gut microbiome's influence on anxiety, mood and depression. "You are what you eat" is such a cliche', but nonetheless true!

Day Fourteen

Gimme that mantra!

_____

_____

How would you rate how you are feeling today? on a scale from 1-10 (10 being off the charts amazing)

① ② ③ ④ ⑤ ⑥ ⑦ ⑧ ⑨ ⑩

_____

If you rated yourself 5 or higher, go get 'em, tiger! See what you can accomplish today! Write those accomplishments down and feel good about it!

If you rated yourself 5 or lower, let's dig in to that.

What is the situation right now occupying your mind?

_____

_____

_____

Are you noticing any physical symptoms? If so, what are they?

_____

_____

_____

_____

Are you noticing any negative thoughts? If so, list them.

_____

_____

_____

_____

Are you able to identify your emotions? (If you are struggling to identify exactly how you are feeling, look at Page 109 to see a list of emotions that we sometimes have difficulty pinpointing.) What emotions are you feeling?

_____

_____

_____

_____

Hit me with those thought stopping techniques and coping skills. Let's take a break, let you catch your breath and jot down some notes about your day if you feel like it.

Notes:

_____

_____

_____

_____

_____

_____

_____

_____

Day Fifteen

You guessed it! Mantra:

_____

_____

How would you rate how you are feeling today? on a scale from 1-10 (10 being off the charts amazing)

① ② ③ ④ ⑤ ⑥ ⑦ ⑧ ⑨ ⑩

_____

Daily Events:

_____

_____

_____

_____

_____

_____

_____

_____

Are you currently, or were you aware of your behavior today?
Was it positive or negative? Explain.

_____

_____

_____

_____

If you found yourself stressy, did you use coping skills? What
coping skills did you use? If you didn't think to use those
skills, what strategies could you have used today? This is a
good way to list them and then remind yourself next time.

_____

_____

_____

_____

Were you able to reframe negative thoughts? Tell me more!
Yes, I sure did and here's how, or no, and explain why.

_____

_____

_____

Were you able to be present? Explain yes or no and why or why not.

_____

_____

_____

_____

What are some thought stopping techniques you used today, or could use in the future?

_____

_____

_____

_____

Let's evaluate the day. How do you think your day ended as opposed to how it started? Rate your recovery from any negative situations 1-10 (10 being amazing and 1 being lousy). If your day started amazing and finished amazing, high five on that 10/10 day! If you found yourself working hard to reframe and recover, high five on doing the work! Rate your day/recovery here:

_____

_____

_____

List three positive things that happened today:

1) _____

2) _____

3) _____

Take some time for yourself today; take a long relaxing bath, get outside and look at some green and blue, or read that book you haven't had time to open! Just 15 minutes can improve your mood!

Day Sixteen

Mantra!

_____

_____

Daily Events:

_____

_____

_____

_____

_____

_____

_____

List the emotions you felt:

_____

_____

_____

If you had a negative emotion, were you able to change your emotion?

If yes, great job! If no, explain why?

_____

_____

_____

_____

If you had a negative emotion and were able to change it, did your behavior change?

_____

_____

_____

_____

Please explain the evidence you uncovered to support your reframe.

_____

_____

_____

_____

After evaluating this situation, on a scale from 1-10 (10 being off the charts amazing), how do you think you did helping yourself?

_____

_____

_____

_____

If you rated how you did with this situation 5 or higher, what did you do that was so effective in helping?

_____

_____

_____

If you rated your handling of the situation 5 or lower, what do you think you could do better next time?

_____

_____

_____

List three positive things that happened today:

1) _____

2) _____

3) _____

Be happy. It drives people crazy.

Day Seventeen

Mantra!

_____

_____

Daily Events:

_____

_____

_____

_____

_____

_____

_____

List the emotions you felt:

_____

_____

_____

If you had a negative emotion, were you able to change your emotion?

If yes, great job! If no, explain why?

_____

_____

_____

_____

If you had a negative emotion and were able to change it, did your behavior change?

_____

_____

_____

_____

Please explain the evidence you uncovered to support your reframe.

_____

_____

_____

_____

After evaluating this situation, on a scale from 1-10 (10 being off the charts amazing), how do you think you did helping yourself?

_____

_____

_____

_____

If you rated how you did with this situation 5 or higher, what did you do that was so effective in helping?

_____

_____

_____

_____

If you rated your handling of the situation 5 or lower, what do you think you could do better next time?

_____

_____

_____

_____

List three positive things that happened today:

1) —————————————————————————

2) —————————————————————————

3) —————————————————————————

"Remember, if you ever need a helping hand, you'll find one at the end of your arm. As you grow older, you will discover you have two hands. One is for helping yourself, the other for helping others."

-Audrey Hepburn

Day Eighteen

Mantra!

_____

_____

Write a little about your day. What was good? What wasn't so good? How did you feel? If we don't write it down, we forget how far we have come! Track your progress!

_____

_____

_____

_____

_____

_____

_____

_____

Did you get some exercise?

_____

What have you eaten today that was good for your body and your soul?

_____

_____

Do you think you will have time to meditate/pray/spend 15 minutes quieting your mind? Write down when this fits in your day, and your pledge to yourself to keep this a priority.

_____

_____

List three positive things that happened today:

1) _____

2) _____

3) _____

*"You can't control what goes on outside, but you CAN control what goes on inside."

-Unknown Author

Day Nineteen

Time to write that mantra!

_____

_____

How would you rate how you are feeling today? on a scale from 1-10 (10 being off the charts amazing)

① ② ③ ④ ⑤ ⑥ ⑦ ⑧ ⑨ ⑩

_____

Daily Events:

_____

_____

_____

_____

_____

_____

_____

Ask yourself what is one thing I can do for myself to move me in a healthy direction. This can be emotionally, mentally, physically or spiritually.

_____

_____

_____

List three positive things that happened today:

1) _____

2) _____

3) _____

Day Twenty

Gimme that mantra!

_____

_____

How would you rate how you are feeling today? on a scale from 1-10 (10 being off the charts amazing)

① ② ③ ④ ⑤ ⑥ ⑦ ⑧ ⑨ ⑩

_____

If you rated yourself 5 or higher, go get 'em, tiger! See what you can accomplish today! Write those accomplishments down and feel good about it!

If you rated yourself 5 or lower, let's dig in to that.

What is the situation right now occupying your mind?

_____

_____

_____

Are you noticing any physical symptoms? If so, what are they?

_____

_____

_____

_____

Are you noticing any negative thoughts? If so, list them.

_____

_____

_____

Are you able to identify your emotions? (If you are struggling to identify exactly how you are feeling, look at Page 109 to see a list of emotions that we sometimes have difficulty pinpointing.) What emotions are you feeling?

_____

_____

_____

_____

Hit me with those thought stopping techniques and coping skills. Let's take a break, let you catch your breath and jot down some notes about your day if you feel like it.

Notes:

_____

_____

_____

_____

_____

_____

_____

_____

_____

_____

Day Twenty-One

You guessed it! Mantra:

_____

_____

How would you rate how you are feeling today? on a scale from 1-10 (10 being off the charts amazing)

① ② ③ ④ ⑤ ⑥ ⑦ ⑧ ⑨ ⑩

_____

Daily Events:

_____

_____

_____

_____

_____

_____

_____

_____

Are you currently, or were you aware of your behavior today?
Was it positive or negative? Explain.

_____

_____

_____

_____

If you found yourself stressy, did you use coping skills? What
coping skills did you use? If you didn't think to use those
skills, what strategies could you have used today? This is a
good way to list them and then remind yourself next time.

_____

_____

_____

_____

Were you able to reframe negative thoughts? Tell me more!
Yes, I sure did and here's how, or no, and explain why.

_____

_____

_____

Were you able to be present? Explain yes or no and why or why not.

What are some thought stopping techniques you used today, or could use in the future?

Let's evaluate the day. How do you think your day ended as opposed to how it started? Rate your recovery from any negative situations 1-10 (10 being amazing and 1 being lousy). If your day started amazing and finished amazing, high five on that 10/10 day! If you found yourself working hard to reframe and recover, high five on doing the work! Rate your day/recovery here:

_____

_____

_____

List three positive things that happened today:

1) _____

2) _____

3) _____

"To keep the body in good health is a duty...otherwise we shall not be able to keep the mind strong and clear."

— Buddha

Day Twenty-Two

Mantra!

_____

_____

Daily Events:

_____

_____

_____

_____

_____

_____

_____

List the emotions you felt:

_____

_____

_____

If you had a negative emotion, were you able to change your emotion?

If yes, great job! If no, explain why?

_____

_____

_____

_____

If you had a negative emotion and were able to change it, did your behavior change?

_____

_____

_____

_____

Please explain the evidence you uncovered to support your reframe.

_____

_____

_____

_____

After evaluating this situation, on a scale from 1-10 (10 being off the charts amazing), how do you think you did helping yourself?

_____

_____

_____

_____

If you rated how you did with this situation 5 or higher, what did you do that was so effective in helping?

_____

_____

_____

If you rated your handling of the situation 5 or lower, what do you think you could do better next time?

_____

_____

_____

_____

List three positive things that happened today:

1) ────────────────────────────

2) ────────────────────────────

3) ────────────────────────────

"The human body has been designed to resist an infinite number of changes and attacks brought about by its environment. The secret of good health lies in successful adjustment to changing stresses on the body."

— Harry J. Johnson

Day Twenty-Three

Mantra!

_____

_____

Daily Events:

_____

_____

_____

_____

_____

_____

_____

List the emotions you felt:

_____

_____

_____

If you had a negative emotion, were you able to change your emotion?

If yes, great job! If no, explain why?

If you had a negative emotion and were able to change it, did your behavior change?

Please explain the evidence you uncovered to support your reframe.

After evaluating this situation, on a scale from 1-10 (10 being off the charts amazing), how do you think you did helping yourself?

_____

_____

_____

_____

If you rated how you did with this situation 5 or higher, what did you do that was so effective in helping?

_____

_____

_____

If you rated your handling of the situation 5 or lower, what do you think you could do better next time?

_____

_____

_____

List three positive things that happened today:

1) _____

2) _____

3) _____

"To help yourself, you must be yourself. Be the best that you can be. When you make a mistake, learn from it, pick yourself up, and move on."

–Unknown Author

Day Twenty-Four

Mantra!

_____

_____

Write a little about your day. What was good? What wasn't so good? How did you feel? If we don't write it down, we forget how far we have come! Track your progress!

_____

_____

_____

_____

_____

_____

_____

Did you get some exercise?

_____

What have you eaten today that was good for your body and your soul?

_____

_____

Do you think you will have time to meditate/pray/spend 15 minutes quieting your mind? Write down when this fits in your day, and your pledge to yourself to keep this a priority.

_____

_____

List three positive things that happened today:

1) _____

2) _____

3) _____

"I have a lot of growing up to do. I realized that the other day inside my fort."

-Zach Galifianakis

Day Twenty-Five

Time to write that mantra!

_____

_____

How would you rate how you are feeling today? on a scale from 1-10 (10 being off the charts amazing)

① ② ③ ④ ⑤ ⑥ ⑦ ⑧ ⑨ ⑩

_____

Daily Events:

_____

_____

_____

_____

_____

_____

_____

_____

Ask yourself what is one thing I can do for myself to move me in a healthy direction. This can be emotionally, mentally, physically or spiritually.

_____

_____

_____

List three positive things that happened today:

1) _____

2) _____

3) _____

Who is your support system? Surround yourself with lovely people who not only want what is best for you, but cheer you on along the way. Remember when your mom told you "you are who you hang around," and you hated it? We hated it too. And then we grew up and saw that the people we spend our time with have a huge impact on us and our mindset. Negativity breeds negativity, and positivity breeds positivity. Toxicity just plain ruins your day. Be picky when it comes to who gets to share your space; you get to choose your tribe.

"Before you marry a person, you should first make them use a computer with slow Internet service to see who they really are."

—Will Ferrell

Day Twenty-Six

You already know-mantra time!

_____

_____

*How would you rate how you are feeling today? on a scale
from 1-10 (10 being off the charts amazing)*

① ② ③ ④ ⑤ ⑥ ⑦ ⑧ ⑨ ⑩

_____

*If you rated yourself 5 or higher, go get 'em, tiger! See what
you can accomplish today! Write those accomplishments
down and feel good about it!*

If you rated yourself 5 or lower, let's dig in to that.

What is the situation right now occupying your mind?

_____

_____

Are you noticing any physical symptoms? If so, what are they?

_____

_____

_____

_____

Are you noticing any negative thoughts? If so, list them.

_____

_____

_____

Are you able to identify your emotions? (If you are struggling to identify exactly how you are feeling, look at Page 109 to see a list of emotions that we sometimes have difficulty pinpointing.) What emotions are you feeling?

_____

_____

_____

_____

Hit me with those thought stopping techniques and coping skills. Let's take a break, let you catch your breath and jot down some notes about your day if you feel like it.

Notes:

_____

_____

_____

_____

_____

_____

_____

_____

_____

_____

Day Twenty-Seven

Time to write that mantra!

_____

_____

How would you rate how you are feeling today? on a scale from 1-10 (10 being off the charts amazing)

① ② ③ ④ ⑤ ⑥ ⑦ ⑧ ⑨ ⑩

_____

Daily Events:

_____

_____

_____

_____

_____

_____

_____

_____

Are you currently, or were you aware of your behavior today? Was it positive or negative? Explain.

_____

_____

_____

_____

If you found yourself stressy, did you use coping skills? What coping skills did you use? If you didn't think to use those skills, what strategies could you have used today? This is a good way to list them and then remind yourself next time.

_____

_____

_____

_____

Were you able to reframe negative thoughts? Tell me more! Yes, I sure did and here's how, or no, and explain why.

_____

_____

_____

Were you able to be present? Explain yes or no and why or why not.

_____

_____

_____

_____

What are some thought stopping techniques you used today, or could use in the future?

_____

_____

_____

_____

Let's evaluate the day. How do you think your day ended as opposed to how it started? Rate your recovery from any negative situations 1-10 (10 being amazing and 1 being lousy). If your day started amazing and finished amazing, high five on that 10/10 day! If you found yourself working hard to reframe and recover, high five on doing the work! Rate your day/recovery here:

_____

_____

_____

List three positive things that happened today:

1) _____

2) _____

3) _____

Remember to keep your humor in life. Not everything is funny, of course; however, if you can find the funny in your day, you will be much better off. Laughter increases your oxygen intake, stimulates the heart and lungs, and increases endorphins, which are stress-relieving hormones. Laughter truly is the best medicine-it's science!

"If you can't make it better, you can laugh at it."

—Erma Bombeck

Day Twenty-Eight

You did it! You made it to day 28! High five!

Mantra!

_____

_____

Daily Events:

_____

_____

_____

_____

_____

_____

_____

List the emotions you felt:

_____

_____

If you had a negative emotion, were you able to change your emotion?

If yes, great job! If no, explain why?

_____

_____

_____

_____

If you had a negative emotion and were able to change it, did your behavior change?

_____

_____

_____

_____

Please explain the evidence you uncovered to support your reframe.

_____

_____

_____

_____

After evaluating this situation, on a scale from 1-10 (10 being off the charts amazing), how do you think you did helping yourself?

_____

_____

_____

_____

If you rated how you did with this situation 5 or higher, what did you do that was so effective in helping?

_____

_____

_____

If you rated your handling of the situation 5 or lower, what do you think you could do better next time?

_____

_____

_____

_____

List three positive things that happened today:

1) ──

2) ──

3) ──

Ok. How do you feel? Do you feel like you benefited from this journaling practice? Take a moment, look back over the last 28 days and think about all that has occurred; have you grown as a person? Do you understand yourself a little better at this point? We sure hope this has been helpful to you. It doesn't have to stop here, of course. Grab a notebook, keep this journal handy and keep going! Don't stop now-you have the tools to keep that positive mindset and make each day better than the last. We are so proud of all your hard work, and for taking the time for yourself. We said it before and we will say it again, you matter. Your health, mental, physical, and spiritual, matters. Ups and downs are promised; it's how you handle them that makes all the difference.

"The unexamined life is not worth living."
— *Socrates*

STRUGGLE BUS

So today is that day; the day that we simply cannot figure this out on our own. Maybe you are overly anxious and cannot get it together. That's ok! You have us! We are going to help you through this.

First, let's talk about grounding techniques. What? What are those? Let's dive in.

Grounding techniques are exercises that can help you focus on the present to put some space between yourself and those anxious feelings you are having. Grounding techniques improve anxiety, reduce stress, and improve your mental well-being. Examples of grounding techniques include but are not limited to the following:

54321 Method: Stop and pay attention to your breathing and heart rate. Take some slow, long, deep breaths. Now, go through the following and list these things either in your head, or out loud, if you feel comfortable.

5 things you can see around you
4 things you can touch
3 things you can hear

2 things you can smell

1 thing you can taste

After doing this, you should feel a certain amount of reduced anxiety, and if your breathing and heart rate were increased, they should be slowing to normal rates. If not, do this exercise again until you start to see improvement in your feelings and physical symptoms.

Memory Game: Look at a photograph or magazine and try to memorize certain things about it. Now look away, and try to recreate that photo or image in your mind. What do you remember about that image? Now go back and see if your memory of it was accurate. Continue to play this game until your anxious feelings improve.

Happy Face, Happy Space: Picture someone you love or someone who makes you feel calm. You can also picture a space that makes you feel happy and relaxed as well. Imagine you are with this person, having a nice beverage and just enjoying each other's company, or imagine occupying that space you love and what you might do there. These thoughts help relax our mind and bring about calmness for us.

Turn That Mutha Down: Imagine your anxiety as having a frequency that can be turned up or down with a dial. Imagine grabbing ahold of that dial and turning that mutha down......all the way down. Turn it down slowly in your head, and breathe deep with each notch. You are making the conscious choice to turn it down, taking control of your feelings and your day.

Listen to Soothing Music: Music is almost magic, isn't it? We can turn on our favorite song and almost instantly change our mood. Classical music has been proven to relax the mind and increase beta-level brain waves. It relieves anxiety and increases problem-solving abilities. Choose whatever music helps you in the moment!

These are just a few examples, but you get the idea. Recite a poem in your head, count to 100, imagine something funny that happened recently; whatever you can do to take your attention and focus away from the negative feeling that's occurring and refocus on something positive.

Situations/Thoughts/Emotions/Behavior

Let's talk about how a thought becomes a behavior.

A situation brings about a thought, right? Let's say you are driving your car and someone pulls out in front of you. Your first thought might be one of fear of having an accident, and your next thought might be "what a jerk!" When you had that jerky thought, you developed an emotion about the situation. Your emotion is a negative one, as you are upset that he/she just paid zero attention and pulled out recklessly. Now, what behavior might you have as a result of that emotion? You might yell, curse, throw your hands in the air in full "what the heck is wrong with you" mode, right? OR WAIT- let's back up to the beginning.

What if, when that person pulled out in front of you, your first thought was, yes, probably still fear at first, but then instead of "what a jerk, your thought was "wow, I hope they are ok! They might be in a hurry for a reason!" This changes your emotion, doesn't it? Now your emotion is one of concern for that person instead of anger. Next, what behavior might you have? It probably isn't going to be yelling and screaming and throwing hands, huh. It might be a kind wave saying 'it's ok, hope you're ok!"

Now, do we know if that person is in a hurry for a good reason or if they are a jerk? No, of course not. But, what happened to you in that moment? Do you feel better or worse after reacting with care and concern over anger? I am going to guess you feel less stressy and more content without the angry feelings. So, does it matter if he/she was a jerk? Not really. How you handle your emotions is what really matters for the sake of yourself and your well-being. So, do you see how a situation brings a thought, a thought brings an emotion, an emotion brings behavior and how we can actually control alllllllll of that? I hope so lol. Hopefully we laid that out well :)

Here are some questions to ask yourself on those struggle bus days. Use the following pages to answer these questions. Refer back to this section as often as you need! This will help you process those situations, thoughts, emotions , and behavior. Take a minute and rate how you are feeling right now on a scale of 1-10, with 1 equalling lousy and 10 equalling amazing. Write it down and write down why.

1. Is there substantial evidence to have this thought?
2. Is there evidence contrary to my thought?
3. Am I attempting to interpret the situation without all of the evidence?

4. What would your friend think about your negative thought?

5. If I look at the situation differently, how is it different?

6. Will this matter in a year? How about five years?

7. Now, what is your reframe?

8. What is the worst-case scenario?

9. What is the best case scenario?

10. What is the most likely case scenario?

Now rate how you feel again, 1-10. Has it improved since you went through this practice? We sure hope so. Keep pushing yourself to see things outside this moment. Stop and think, if a friend brought me this problem, how would I see it for them versus how I see it for myself? We are usually way harder on ourselves than we should be. Keep up the good, hard work! You are so worth it!

Vocabulary of Emotions

Confusion	Sad	Strong	Happy	Anger	Energized
Uncertain	Depressed	Sure	Amused	Annoyed	Determined
Upset	Desperate	Certain	Delighted	Agitated	Inspired
Doubtful	Dejected	Unique	Glad	Fed Up	Creative
Indecisive	Heavy	Dynamic	Pleased	Irritated	Healthy
Perplexed	Crushed	Tenacious	Charmed	Mad	Renewed
Embarrassed	Disgusted	Hardy	Grateful	Critical	Vibrant
Hesitant	Upset	Secure	Optimistic	Resentful	Strengthened
Shy	Hateful	Empowered	Content	Outraged	Motivated
Lost	Sorrowful	Ambitious	Joyful	Furious	Focused
Unsure	Mournful	Powerful	Enthusiastic	Livid	Invigorated
Pessimistic	Weepy	Confident	Loving	Bitter	Refreshed
Tense	Frustrated	Determined	Marvelous	Irrational	Excited

Emotion Exploration Scale

Emotion Exploration Scale

Understanding what an emotion feels like, and how it changes as it grows, is one of the first steps to learning how to control the emotion. Choose an emotion you would like to explore and describe how it progresses from the lowest possible level (1) to the highest possible level (10).

1	2	3	4	5	6	7	8	9	10

Emotion:

Thoughts

Behaviors

Symptoms / Physical Sensations

Thoughts

Behaviors

Symptoms / Physical Sensations

Thoughts

Behaviors

Symptoms / Physical Sensations

Gratitude Exercises

Gratitude means appreciating the good things in life, no matter how big or small. Making the practice of gratitude a regular part of your day can build happiness, self-esteem, and provide other health benefits.

Gratitude Journal

Every evening, spend a few minutes writing down some good things about your day. This isn't limited to major events. You might be grateful for simple things, such as a good meal, talking to a friend, or overcoming an obstacle.

Give Thanks

Keep your eyes open throughout the day for reasons to say "thank you." Make a conscious effort to notice when people do good things, whether for you or others. Tell the person you recognize their good deed, and give a sincere "thank you."

Mindfulness Walk

Go for a walk and make a special effort to appreciate your surroundings. You can do this by focusing on each of your senses, one at a time. Spend a minute just listening, a minute looking at your surroundings, and so on. Try to notice the sights, sounds, smells, and sensations you would usually miss, such as a cool breeze on your skin, or the clouds in the sky.

Gratitude Letter

Think about someone who you appreciate. This could be a person who has had a major impact on your life, or someone who you would like to thank. Write a letter that describes why you appreciate them, including specific examples and details. It's up to you if you'd like to share the letter or not.

Grateful Contemplation

Remove yourself from distractions such as phones or TV and spend 5-10 minutes mentally reviewing the good things from your day. The key to this technique is *consistency*. Think of it like brushing your teeth or exercise—it should be a normal part of daily self-care. This technique can be practiced as part of prayer, meditation, or on its own.

Gratitude Conversation

With another person, take turns listing 3 things you were grateful for throughout the day. Spend a moment discussing and contemplating each point, rather than hurrying through the list. Make this part of your routine by practicing before a meal, before bed, or at another regular time.

Provided by **TherapistAid.com**

Urge Surfing Script-1

Urge Surfing
guided meditation script

Urge surfing is a technique for managing your unwanted behaviors. While practicing, you will ride out an urge, like a surfer riding a wave.

brief pause ────────────────────────────

Sit back or lie down in a comfortable position. Close your eyes, or let your gaze soften.

brief pause ────────────────────────────

Much like an ocean wave, an urge will gradually gain strength, peak, and then fade away.

brief pause ────────────────────────────

When an urge is growing or at its peak, it often feels as if it will never go away. You might feel discomfort, or like you *have to* act on the urge. Remember, these are just feelings.

brief pause ────────────────────────────

Notice where you are on the wave of your urge. Is the urge gaining strength, peaking, or beginning to fade?

20-30 second pause ────────────────────────────

Remind yourself that urges are temporary. No matter how intense your urge, it will eventually weaken and disappear, even if you don't act upon it.

10 second pause ────────────────────────────

The goal of urge surfing isn't to change your thoughts and feelings. Instead, you will try to accept whatever you are experiencing.

brief pause ────────────────────────────

Take a moment to notice your thoughts. Simply observe the words or images in your mind.

30-45 second pause ────────────────────────────

Shift your attention to your feelings. You might have uncomfortable feelings, such as anger, temptation, or guilt. Even uncomfortable feelings are okay.

30-45 second pause ────────────────────────────

Urge Surfing
guided meditation script

Now we will practice a relaxation technique called visualization. This will help you continue to ride out your urge.

brief pause

Use all your senses to imagine the following scene.

brief pause

Imagine you're standing on a beautiful, sandy beach. You feel the warmth of the sun on your face, and a gentle breeze on your skin.

15-25 second pause

You begin to walk slowly down the shore. With each step, the sand crunches beneath your feet.

15-25 second pause

Birds sing in the distance, and ocean waves rumble steadily along the shore.

15-25 second pause

You take a step toward the ocean and stand at the edge of the surf. Cool water rushes over the top of your feet.

15-25 second pause

The air is warm, and smells salty.

15-25 second pause

You look out toward the ocean and notice the water contains every shade of blue and green. When the waves peak, they shimmer in the sunlight, before disappearing onto the shore.

30 second pause

You continue standing on the shore, taking in the sensations of the beach, the ocean, and the waves.

60-90 second pause

Urge Surfing
guided meditation script

The waves in the ocean are just like your urge. They are powerful for a short time, but before long they peak, and then fade away. You don't have to suppress your urge or try to change it. It will simply fade away on its own.

brief pause ─────────────────────────

Now, begin to focus on your breathing. For the next few minutes, you'll practice taking slow, deep breaths, which will help reduce stress and anxiety.

brief pause ─────────────────────────

You'll inhale for 4 seconds, hold the air in your lungs for 4 seconds, then slowly exhale for 6 seconds.

When inhaling, focus on completely filling your lungs with air.

brief pause ─────────────────────────

To start, follow along as I walk you through the breathing cycle. Let's begin:

brief pause ─────────────────────────

Inhale, 2, 3, 4

Hold, 2, 3, 4

Exhale, 2, 3, 4, 5, 6

Inhale, 2, 3, 4

Hold, 2, 3, 4

Exhale, 2, 3, 4, 5, 6

Inhale

3 second pause ─────────────────────────

Hold

3 second pause ─────────────────────────

Exhale

5 second pause ─────────────────────────

3

Urge Surfing
guided meditation script

Inhale

3 second pause ————————————————————————————

Hold

3 second pause ————————————————————————————

Exhale

5 second pause ————————————————————————————

Continue practicing on your own for a few minutes.

60-90 second pause ————————————————————————

During deep breathing, it's normal for your mind to wander. When you notice this happening, simply return your attention to your breathing, noticing how it feels to take slow, deep breaths.

120-180 second pause ————————————————————————

This exercise is nearly complete. Before continuing your day, take one more moment to observe your thoughts and feelings. Notice if your urge has changed.

30-45 second pause ————————————————————————

When you feel ready to do so, open your eyes and stretch.

15 second pause ————————————————————————————

This concludes the urge surfing exercise. If you'd like to continue practicing, you can start the exercise again, as many times as you need.

The Cognitive Triangle

The Cognitive Triangle

The **cognitive triangle** shows how thoughts, emotions, and behaviors affect one another. This means changing your *thoughts* will change how you *feel and behave*.

A **situation** is anything that happens in your life, which triggers the cognitive triangle.

Thoughts are your interpretations of a situation. For example, if a stranger looks at you with an angry expression, you could think: "Oh no, what did I do wrong?" or "Maybe they are having a bad day."

Emotions are feelings, such as happy, sad, angry, or worried. Emotions can have physical components as well as mental, such as low energy when feeling sad, or a stomachache when nervous.

Behaviors are your response to a situation. Behaviors include actions such as saying something or doing something (or, choosing not to do something).

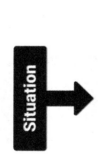

Situation → **Thoughts** ↔ **Emotions** ↔ **Behaviors**

Provided by **TherapistAid.com**

Coping Skills
Depression

Behavioral Activation

Depression saps a person's energy to do just about anything—even activities they enjoy. As a result, people with depression tend to become less active, which causes the depression to worsen. However, even a little bit of activity can help stop this cycle.

1. Choose activities you are likely to complete.

exercise	walk, go for a bike ride, weightlift, follow an exercise video, swim, practice yoga
socialize	call or text a friend, organize a group dinner, visit family, join a club / group
responsibilities	cleaning / housework, pay bills, professional development, homework
hobbies	sports, gardening, drawing, playing music, hiking, playing with a pet, cooking
personal care	dress up, get a haircut, prepare a healthy meal, tend to spiritual needs

2. Practice your chosen activities. Use the following tips to improve consistency.

start small	If needed, break activities into smaller pieces. Some activity is better than none.
make a plan	Set an alarm as a reminder, or tie an activity to something you already do. For example, practice a hobby immediately after dinner every day.
bring a friend	Including a friend will increase your commitment and make things more fun.

Social Support

Social isolation is a common symptom of depression. Related issues—such as fatigue, lowered self-esteem, and anxiety—exacerbate this problem. Resisting social isolation, and instead leaning on social support, can improve resilience to stress and depression.

✓ **Lean on your existing relationships.** Make it a priority to socialize with friends or family every day. If this is proving difficult, or if no one is nearby, plan times to interact remotely. Try cooking together on a video call, playing a game together, or sharing a coffee over the phone.

✓ **Say "yes" to socializing.** Depression makes it tempting to stay home, isolated from friends and family. Make a habit of saying "yes" to social opportunities, even when you're tempted to stay in.

✓ **Join a support group.** Support groups let you connect with others who are dealing with issues similar to yours. You'll benefit from sharing and receiving advice and support.

Coping Skills
Depression

Three Good Things

Negative thinking is a defining feature of depression. Positive experiences are minimized, while negative experiences are magnified. Gratitude helps combat this tendency by shifting focus toward *positive* experiences, rather than negative ones.

1 Write about three positive experiences from your day. These experiences can be small ("The weather was perfect when I walked to work") or big ("I got a promotion at work").

2 Choose one of the following questions to answer about each of the three good things:
- Why did this happen?
- Why was this good thing meaningful?
- How can I experience more of this good thing?

3 Repeat this exercise every day for 1 week.

Mindfulness

Mindfulness means paying attention to the present moment. It means taking a step back and noticing the world, and one's thoughts and feelings, without judgment. The goal of mindfulness is to simply *observe*. Mindfulness helps reduce the rumination and worry that often accompany depression.

One way to practice mindfulness is through meditation. During mindfulness meditation, you will simply sit and focus your attention on the sensation of breathing. By focusing on your breathing, you will put yourself in the here-and-now.

🕐 Time and Place
Find a quiet, comfortable place where you can practice mindfulness for 15 to 30 minutes every day. Frequent and consistent practice leads to the best results, but some practice is better than none.

🪑 Posture
Sit in a chair or lie down in a comfortable position. Close your eyes or let your gaze soften. Let your head, shoulders, arms, and legs relax. Adjust your posture whenever you feel uncomfortable.

🌬 Awareness of Breath
Focus on your breathing. Notice the sensation of the air as it travels in through your nose and out through your mouth. Notice the gentle rise and fall of your belly.

🪧 Wandering Mind
During meditation, it's normal for the mind to wander. When this happens, gently turn your attention back to your breathing. You may need to do this frequently throughout your practice.

Reference

Rodriguez, T (2013).Write to heal. Scientific American Mind, 24 (5), p. 17. doi:10.1038/scientificamericanmind1113-17b

Worksheets courtesy of *therapistaid.com*. Therapistaid.com is a wonderful service offering many features at no charge.
https://www.therapistaid.com/therapy-worksheets?page=5

You've Got the POWER

CHOOSE YOUR SHINE

small steps every day

be the BEST version of you

YOU'RE-DOING Great

POSITIVE MIND

Believe in Yourself

I am capable

you're AMAZING

-STAY- POSITIVE

SMILE everyday

yes you can

FOCUS ON THE GOOD

GOOD VIBES

clean your MIND

FOLLOW YOUR HEART

BE Bold

you are loved

You Got This!

TREAT yourself

Proud OF myself

be happy

CHASE Goals

be Brave

you're LOVED

Kindness MATTERS

Made in the USA
Columbia, SC
28 November 2022

72057905R00070